ISAIAH'S

A MOTHER'S FIRST YEAR JOURNEY WITH A BABY BORN AT 23 WEEKS

CHAPTER

Ebony Horton

Isaiah's Chapter
A Mother's First Year Journey With A Baby Born At 23 Weeks

Scriptures taken from the Holy Bible, New International Version®, NIV®. Copyright © 1973, 1978, 1984 by Biblica, Inc.™ Used by permission of Zondervan. All rights reserved worldwide.www.zondervan.com.

ISBN: 0988266903
ISBN-13: 978-0-9882669-0-2

DEDICATION

This book is dedicated to God. Without His pushing and His blessing in Isaiah, this book would not exist. Jelan and Isaiah, this is also for you. Without your brown eyes full of hope, without the clinch of your small hands when a tube prevented you from cooing, and without your unconditional love, this project could never have reached beyond my little diary. The joy you've brought will never be forgotten. I love you.

CONTENT

Special thanks to ...

Grandma Josephine, for your patience and care for Isaiah as I wrote his story for others to share,

My mom, Alicia, my aunt, Deborah, Isaiah's godparents, Sam and Reba Hall, and the rest of my family for your mental support and for enduring with me the trials of a hospital stay,

Amanda, Nancy and Tammy, for your love for Isaiah, music and books while he underwent consistent and often painful treatments,

The March of Dimes, for its countless resources and efforts to curb premature childbirth,

The Ronald McDonald House staff for your encouraging words and immeasurable hospitality, and

Lastly, but certainly not least, friends Jerick Cooper, Macie Holloway, Julia Sanders and Artez Jones for your assistance and your wisdom through this process.

INTRODUCTION

I'VE OFTEN SAID I don't know what it's like to birth a healthy baby or to hold my newborn after the very first cry. I do, however, know what it is to have a miracle child.

My oldest son lived almost three months on oxygen between an incubator and crib in a neonatal intensive care unit after he was born at just 26 weeks' gestation. He went through the pneumonia, the infections, the painkillers and much else that even some adults couldn't survive. Yet even through this process, I don't ever recall a moment of losing hope while on the "roller coaster" of medical prognoses and physical distress.

With Isaiah, both my life and my logic were different than the first time around. Because I had unknowingly dilated around two centimeters at only 23 weeks, doctors believed Isaiah had only a 13-percent chance of existing beyond his fetal state. If he did survive, it was likely he would live only a couple days. It seemed I chose this pregnancy to believe the doctors over my Savior, so I lost hope. My family thought they had lost me.

We all have a tendency to block out parts of the tragedies we face so we don't have to relive what we suffered when the incident first occurred. But I have since learned that sometimes, it's necessary to tell our story for the next person who might have to endure but who is unable at some point to see the light at the end of the tunnel.

I knew from the beginning of Isaiah's life that there was something about his story that needed to be shared with more than just our inner circle. So, I logged my experiences with my child in more than just a diary and a scrapbook. I wrote of his life through weekly letters to my co-workers and friends.

Here is one of the first letters that began our travels in life. Others are intertwined in the chapters ahead:

April 22, 2009
Subject: My miracle, and you

Dear family,

I delivered at 23 weeks and after three doctors said Isaiah Samuel would not survive
before 24 weeks, yet another doctor came and said my baby's heart was not beating outside of my body.
But in just seconds, all of that changed.
Isaiah is three days old, is drinking milk, and is working toward breathing on his own. Doctors found none of the bleeding in his precious brain that is typically associated to premature birth, and his one and a half-pound body is fully formed.
He is hooked up to quite a bit of equipment at the hospital and has some growing to do. Yet I believe these moments are tied into God's plan for us and that Isaiah will come out of this whole, healthy and strong.
While his journey isn't over, I pray that each of you know I am so grateful for all you have done and all you have been in this time for us.
You are the heartbeat of my hope. Even when things don't go as expected, I know I'm never without your prayers that we will make it through. Many people will never be blessed with such a strong web of friends, family and coworkers.
Thank you for everything. You are never without my prayers.

Ebony

With the prayers of those who were strong when I couldn't have been, and with a God who knows everything that I thought I didn't, we shared a full first year with a living being. You'll discover in this book how Isaiah's name alone was a promise of his destiny.

I'm humbled, honored, and hopeful for this opportunity to tell a portion of Isaiah's chapter in my life. My prayer is that you find as much peace and encouragement as I did in the joy experienced after testing through Isaiah's first year.

Please keep in mind this book is simply a story of our personal journey. It is not intended to provide medical advice, diagnosis or treatment.

~~~~~~~~~~~~~~~~~~~**1**~~~~~~~~~~~~~~~~

AGAIN

"So do not fear, for I am with you; do not be dismayed, for I am your God. I will strengthen you and help you; I will uphold you with my righteous right hand."

Isaiah 41:10

SOMETIMES, WE MAY take healthy children for granted. Many of us don't know what it's like to see an innocent child fight for his life, and we squawk at the need to take days off work to tend to a baby's small cough or fever. But perspectives tend to change when symptoms of the simplest ailments turn severe, or when you're praying to hear your baby's heartbeat again.

I've been there twice.

Both my boys were born far less than two pounds each and not breathing, and both spent months in hospitals that were hours away from where we lived.

I've felt the anxiety, fear, anger and blame at a time I should have been smiling to hear "It's a boy!" or "Girl." I still covet the moment I should have been calling to give the color of his eyes and brag on the natural delivery in inches and pounds of a bouncing newborn son.

Those hopes shattered in a hospital bed on a morning that was months before the time Isaiah was supposed to arrive.

I thought whatever needed to be fixed was taken care of the first time, the first trauma I had three hours from home when a doctor woke me from a medically induced sleep to tell me my first son had a 50-percent chance of survival after he would likely come at 26 weeks' gestation.

I knew this baby was going to make it, however. We had just decided on a name, which meant "Mighty Faith," and we were expecting the blessing that had been "cooking in the oven" for six months, despite the three-month shortcut around my last trimester.

Indeed, faith and a merciful God paid off.

Yes, Jelan Iman (Jey-lahn Ih-mahn) came without breathing. I stopped breathing for a while, too, and the next time we saw each other, Jelan was in a rectangular, clear box they called an incubator with tubes all around him and a light that showed the tiny veins running through his one-pound, nine-ounce frame.

But all the fingers and toes were there. That's the first thing most people seem to look for. Everything actually was fully formed. We could see his ribs, his heartbeat and all else through his frail skin.

Some of the prognoses were scary. All the brain bleed or intraventricular hemorrhage (IVH) conversation, breathing issues, pneumonia and early intervention talks would plague us for a full three months of going to a neonatal intensive care unit (or NICU) to visit our baby. We had to read to him through that box because we couldn't hold him. When we did hold him, it could only be done with proper supervision.

Jelan came home in November 2005 to the promises that Mommy would do absolutely everything in her power to assure he'd have the best life possible, despite discussions that he could very well be developmentally impaired. Still, he was beautiful. He grew so fast to become a toddler, and thank God he was fine despite a couple breathing issues early on. We still had no idea why he was born premature but related it to the potential stress of having a first child during my busy schedule as a writer and English student.

There was no inclination that I would experience a premature birth again, and three years would pass before the morning sickness returned. This time, I was going to play things safely and hope for a better turnout. I was prescribed steroids as a precaution in hopes of strengthening my uterus and my baby in case of an early labor. I tried to take it as easy as possible.

"As easy as possible" still didn't work. The likelihood of potential tragedy hit again on what should have been yet another great day in my life – the day we would discover whether we were having a girl or a boy.

A Second

"Come on in Miss Horton" were the words the obstetrician gynecologist's nurse faintly said as Jelan accompanied Mommy to her appointment. Those words were spoken from the same woman I'd almost approached for her unwelcoming spirit on several occasions. But something was different that day. She could have said she hated me and still would have been greeted with as large of a smile as she was with her coarse welcome. "Okay, thanks!" I yelled. Jelan and I were about to hear the greatest news we had in a long time, albeit Mommy's cramps were strong and I was tired from a night's work. We were about to find out what we were having!

We went in for the sonogram and sure enough, it was another boy. My heart jumped as Jelan called Daddy, but the high dropped suddenly when my doctor called me into his office. I felt my spirits dampen and my hands press together at the sound of the news that I had prayed could not be possible.

"The baby is a little lower than he should be at 20 weeks."
"Oh that's fine," I said. "The old tales are they are low when they are boys. When is our next visit?"
"Well, you're going to have to stay here a while."
"Stay where a while?"
"In the hospital. You're at risk of having this one early, too. I'm so sorry, but at 20 weeks, your baby will not make it."
"Will not make what?"

There we had it – more negativity before anything good. This time, though, I was more moved to buy the doctor's words than the faith I had tuned in to on a regular basis when we heard similar news at Jelan's birth.

Family came and picked up Jelan as an ambulance transported me to a hospital four hours away. I was to lie upside down in a bed for a few weeks trying to keep Isaiah inside for just a little longer. As medically advanced as the world had gotten, tilting a pregnant woman in hopes of gravity working a baby back inside seemed a bit ancient, but I was willing to do anything I could to keep the child alive. According to the doctor, a baby had around a 13-percent chance of survival if he made it to 24 weeks gestation, which he said was medically accepted as the earliest that a baby could live outside of the mother's belly. Any period below 24 weeks was declared heavily opportune for a miscarriage, so if Isaiah wouldn't wait, we thought he wouldn't live. I had already dilated two centimeters.

The doctors at the larger hospital were able to insert a pessary or a sort of ring to support my uterus because Isaiah had dropped too low for my uterus to be surgically sewn, so fortunately Isaiah was brought back home in his mommy's belly still breathing. We were to be on bed rest, but I guess Isaiah didn't like the idea because at 22 weeks and six days, my water broke. I believed the doctor when he said my baby wouldn't live, so instead of going to the hospital that was a half-hour away because the local one didn't deliver babies, I just drove around. I cried with my mother over the phone and tried to enjoy what I thought would be the last few bonding moments with my child before burying him forever. I mustered up enough nerve to call the doctor who disclosed the first bad news and asked if I could go to the local hospital and wait for a doctor to come and remove my child.

It was the same doctor who told me the baby would die who attempted to calm my steady flow of tears and convince me to take the drive. He promised to contact the doctors at the hospital four hours away after examining how low Isaiah had pushed through. After I made the drive, there was a little relief when another one of those mentally torturing uterus exams showed Isaiah had not come down any lower than the two centimeters from two weeks ago. The doctor said the staff at the other hospital believed there was still a possibility Isaiah could grow inside of me for another couple weeks because at 26 weeks, there would be a 50-percent chance he would live. So, the doctor decided to have me transported. The only problem was that with my water broken, Isaiah was losing the necessary fluid to prevent infection.

~~~~~~~~~~~~~~~~~~~~~**2**~~~~~~~~~~~~~~~~~~~

FROM THE FIRST HEARTBEAT

" ...The Lord is the everlasting God, the Creator of the ends of the earth.
... Even youths grow tired and weary, and young men stumble and fall;
but those who hope in the Lord will renew their strength. They will soar
on wings like eagles; they will run and not grow weary, they will walk
and not be faint. "

Isaiah 40:28, 30-31

NAMES ARE OF significant meaning in my family. We've never been ones to create them. We always attempt to pass them down the family line, or to discover new namesakes with biblical roots or those that are encouraging in nature.

We'd thought there were at least three more months to ponder a name for the newest addition to our family, but after returning home and having to be transported again to a hospital four hours away from my home, my body had become infected. I thought a name was useless, but the Biblical book Isaiah – along with its promises of healing and a Savior – came to mind.

I had never read the book all the way through. I promised that I would, seeing that I believed somewhere in there was some kind of guarantee that the baby inside of me would be alright. I determined that if there was a promise there, then I would name the child Isaiah, and pray – as the name meant – that the Lord would "help me." I lay again with my feet propelled in the air. I had gained my faith again and started the prayers rolling. I was going to have another sweet baby boy! The second joy of my life was a little more excited to meet us than we wanted him to be, but things had gotten back on schedule and he would see us in a few weeks. I was pumped with steroids and magnesium sulfate in hopes of developing his lungs in case he still decided to come early, but with a pessary and the upside down position, it was possible he could even make it halfway into the third trimester.

A working mother, I wondered how long Isaiah would "cook" inside the oven and how long the rest of my life could do without me. Hopes were that Isaiah would not come for another couple weeks, so I had to figure how to balance the remainder of my six weeks leave from work if I were to technically spend two of them in labor. I knew immediate child care was not the answer, so I focused on tweeting about being inside the hospital and penned other ideas in a diary to keep my mind off my post-delivery plans. The first day of this newfound time occupation went well. With family so far away, there were really no visitors on the second stay besides my college friend Julia, who lived about thirty minutes away. We chatted about our futures and her "nephew" a few short minutes before nightfall, when I first noticed blood in the bathroom. Of course, these issues had to occur at a shift change, and the nurse brushed things off as "normal."

Next thing I know, nurses transported me off an emergency floor to a room in a maternal ward that appeared to be more of a home setting. I hugged my friend goodbye and settled in as if I would be there for days. That's when the cramps hit. A resident doctor warned me that the cramps were a sure sign of infection of the amniotic fluid in which the baby dwelled. Any such infection, called chorioamnionitis, could potentially kill both Isaiah and me. I couldn't wrap my mind around how I had almost lost Isaiah once and was facing the grief cycle a second time in just 48 short hours. Nonetheless, the shivers came, and it was not long before I was transferred to labor and delivery so that doctors could induce the labor.

The Delivery

I don't remember much about the labor pains other than trouble using the bathroom and begging nurses not to insert another catheter. I do, however, remember the unforgettable feeling of the little foot of my little one pressing through to try to save himself.

We delivered naturally on the morning of April 19, 2009. At 23 weeks and one day, Isaiah was one pound and five ounces and around six inches. He had no heartbeat and gave no cry. In one moment, a doctor said, "Miss Horton, we are trying, but I don't think your baby is going to make it." That's when I nodded. Maybe it just was meant to be.

Alone – away from family whose jobs had prevented long term stays with me in a city so far from our houses – I was to bear the news that I had lost a child. I somehow was to call everyone and say that Isaiah was gone and we were to arrange for a funeral. I created a mental list of who to call first, and which loved one to assign to call the others. I didn't know whether to text or to ring my editor so that he could spread the news. I tweeted the few-minute delivery of my baby, but I didn't know how to message that he died. I hoped the phone would die, too, so I wouldn't have the responsibility.

In the corner of the room, experienced neonatal nurses still attempted to get my baby to respond. I wished they would stop trying and quit pressuring a dead body to cry. I had already taken the doctor's word again without my own research, and every sound from the opposite side of the room where they were working just gave me what I thought was more false hope. I wondered how I could ever have believed Isaiah would make it. How dare I put my family through this again? How dare I pray for a healthy baby and promise the bundle in the belly that things would be okay? Why did I make plans and envision the child growing older and smiling with me about how God had brought him through?

I looked to the ceiling a final time before closing my eyes in exhaustion.

Then, a miracle happened.

"Miss Horton," another voice said much softer than the one of the doctor. "Look here at your baby. He is beautiful, and he is fine. We are going to take him away for a while, but you can come see him soon."

I'd lost a lot of blood and was barely alert, so I don't know if I gave a sigh of relief or a sigh of fear that history would repeat itself.

But, from that very first heartbeat, I knew it was a journey we would all take together.

~~~~~~~~~~~~~~~~~~~~**3**~~~~~~~~~~~~~~~~~~~~

TWO DAYS OF LIFE

"Listen to me ... you whom I have upheld since you were conceived, and have carried since your birth. Even to your old age and gray hairs I am he, I am he who will sustain you. I have made you and I will carry you; I will sustain you and I will rescue you."

Isaiah 46:3-4

THE INTERNING DOCTORS said if your premature baby makes it past the first 48 hours, you're generally good. So there was hope after all! "He's actually breathing on his own," one doctor said when I laid eyes on my baby for the first time.

Isaiah lay greased on a white sheet. He was, indeed, breathing on his own. His tiny little one-pound body was fully formed, and his chest was going up and down. His head was covered with slick, black hair, and his arms and legs lay stretched out as if he was just taking a long nap. He wouldn't open his eyes, but I didn't care. I didn't know what it was like to call in eye colors, anyway. I only knew what it was like to say the baby was alive and to solicit prayers from everyone I knew.

Even with the tiny tubes needed to initially assist him into life, Isaiah was one of the most gorgeous babies I had ever seen. And there was one good sign after another. Although it would take a couple days to get results back, there were no initial symptoms of internal bleeding. Really, that message of hope was all I needed to keep my spirits high. After carrying another baby for as many months before, the last thing you want to know is that he might have to fight harder than you did. Any sign of relief from a doctor was always good to me.

Just as disheartening, though, is a sign of fear, and I'm sure most all families of premature infants know of the "roller coaster" in which doctors warn. There are the high moments, but you might also expect a low one to come soon. In a NICU you can never – so they say – keep high spirits on a continual basis. You have to fit time in your schedule to take in the possibilities of the worst, even when your baby is well.

The First Diagnoses

It seemed like just minutes between the time Isaiah went from breathing on his own and having all his organs fully developed to him suffering the next to worst severe brain hemorrhaging that there was, which was known as a Grade 3. He was suffering from sepsis, or a variety of blood infections, and apnea (severe difficulty in catching his own breath or breathing regularly), and he was susceptible to multiple viruses and blood infections. It was, as the doctor had said, a full 48 hours of bliss before the tests and the trauma on my baby's body started setting in again. As most premature babies, he needed blood transfusions to survive because he couldn't make blood fast enough. With Type O blood, the bank for the transfusions was rare. He needed a ventilator to help him stay alive, yet he was jittery so it was hard for nurses to keep the tube down his throat in the right position. Water also surrounded his brain in a condition known as Hydrocephalus.

He would soon start having seizures and he needed sedatives multiple times throughout the day. He began losing an ounce here and an ounce there. He developed jaundice and several bacterial and viral infections because his body was too weak for both the fight and the medication. The toes on his left foot had blackened, likely because of a low blood circulation flow. Some doctors believed the toes were gangrenous. No matter how medically advanced the doctors were, the results of multiple tests still took time. So we would get the result of one test, and find out that our baby was suffering from even more.

One thing that was stressed, though, was breast milk, and the benefit was that Isaiah was eating the milk I pumped daily one little millileter at a time. Apparently a mother's breast milk has natural antibodies designed specifically for the child, and Isaiah needed every little ounce that Mommy could get to him. "We can only hope he doesn't get the types of infections that could be deadly, but your baby is very, very sick, and you were too," the doctor said. "The breast milk is one of the best things you can do for your baby. Other than that, you have to just hope for the best."

Your mind starts seeing and selectively hearing after a series of bad news. All I could hear was "sick," a repeat of the 50-percent chance of living for my first child. But, his heart was beating. There had to be something good to come out of that. I just knew that no matter how sick I was, no matter how much blood I lost, I had to be there for Isaiah and Jelan. I asked God to cover me, to help me get through. I was going to have to survive somehow, because I was about to enter yet another fight of life.

Isaiah was already in the ring. There he would be, frantically hoping for rest from the constant pricking and testing he had to endure. The point, however, was that he was there, ready for whatever was necessary to get him home. I was, too.

4

FIGHTING ALONE

"Those who are wayward in spirit will gain understanding; ...Be our strength every morning, our salvation in time of distress."

Isaiah 29:24; 33:2

THERE ARE THE perks to living in a small, semi-country town in southeastern Alabama. You have fewer traffic jams, and – whether you consider it a plus or a minus – everyone knows each other by name. Your church family is unified and your friends hear more about you than you tell. Your biological family is usually down the street from each other on a road named after an ancestor, and everyone is familiar with the graces – and misfortunes – of your family line.

But, there are the negatives. One big one is that when you have a premature child, at least when I did in 2009, the nearest medical hubs that can care for you are at least three hours away in a much, much larger city. That means the close-knit family, the church groups and traffic jams are three hours away, too, so much of your battle is tasked with the fear of fighting alone. So you're faced with two choices. Be lonely or mingle. I chose, after about three days of total loneliness, to mingle.

It was through these interactions with nurses and other parents that I learned Isaiah and me would probably both be at the hospital for quite some time. While a surviving 23-weeker was rare, there were children born after 24 weeks whose families lived as far as we had. We needed somewhere to live, and it appeared business owners both for profit and not-for-profit were prepared for our circumstances. We called several places, some that charged, some that didn't. We ultimately ended up in a Ronald McDonald House.

There, you don't ask how people are. You nod and you smile. If you get a nod or a smile back, you ask about their baby. If you don't, you say a prayer, because that usually means things aren't well. Staff at the house doesn't force you to talk, either. There's a set time to eat and a few moments to fellowship. But it's not required.

Staying with the 'Family'

You never know what life-altering changes one has made until you interact with the other families. I learned from Donna and Merck that they left home and jobs in a southeastern Alabama town four hours away to be with their little miracle child. They'd been at the house five months, but after five other miscarriages, the couple was willing to do anything to watch their sweet 26-weeker with green eyes make it through.

I met other couples whose children were just there for checkups and had to be monitored over a period of time. There was the single mom with two other kids who trekked up and down the hospital stairs to see about their little one. There was also another mother that I met during a sort of support group meeting at the hospital. She ironically was from the same city as me, and our encounters would become far more common than I would have imagined.

One family's baby had thrived for a week or so before one of her lungs collapsed. After our first greeting and agreement to pray for each other, I never saw her again at the house.

I walked back and forth between the hospital and house trying to focus on only Isaiah and our situation, but the thought that others were doing better or worse always bothered me over the first two weeks. You might understand my joy then when I learned my neighbor in the house was the mother of the baby next to Isaiah in the NICU. That baby was born at 23 weeks and four days. Isaiah had been born at 23 weeks and one day, but it appeared both the babies had similar issues. While the mother and father didn't talk much, it was reassuring that my struggle was not the only of its kind.

Staying in the NICU

From my experience with Jelan as a premature baby, I knew that books and music were highly recommended, so I invested in some childrens' books and some classical music CDs, as well as brought some Gospel music CDs that had been given to Jelan. I played the music in Isaiah's little headphones around the clock and tried my best to keep batteries available and to be on hand to turn the CD when necessary. I made it a point to be in the hospital around the time each doctor made his rounds, and tried my best to comb through answers in the doctors' generic responses. Things weren't the best, but they were looking like survival as we approached Isaiah's first month in the NICU. I even got to hold him for a few minutes while he was wrapped tightly in warm blankets and wore a hat. He was no bigger than my forearm, but he was warm and he was breathing, albeit with a ventilator. He still didn't attempt to see me, but in my heart, I knew he felt my presence and wanted me there.

I spent time researching premature infancy and every study I could find that pertained to 23-weekers. Unfortunately, there was minimal literature on the topic because so many in Isaiah's situation had passed on before research could take place. That lone fact was basically the reason I felt led by God to write this book. My son's life was truly a miracle.

I continued pumping the breast milk as many times throughout the day as I could. The remainder of the time, I stood by my baby's side and de-stressed with e-mails to my family and co-workers. They supported me both by prayer and finances to assure I had little to nothing to worry about but my child. One letter sounded like this:

May 8, 2009
Subject: Isaiah Week Three

Isaiah's third week was up and down, but mostly up. We had some respiratory issues toward the end and a couple mild run-ins with nurses, who kind of rushed to medicate before taking all other measures. But I was professional, and learned more about assertiveness and trusting God for action. Isaiah stayed weighed in at about two pounds over the week. I'm getting to hold him more. The brain bleeding was absorbing some and we were having no problems with eating from the tube at all. Most of what he was going through we endured with Jelan, so I truly know Isaiah is going to be fine.

It's at those times of bliss, though, that the nurses remind you of the emotional roller coaster and that things won't always be as well as they were at first. I had to learn to adjust to the nurses' philosophy every time I heard a buzzer sound off that alerted them of my baby's dropped heart rate or fast breathing with the ventilator. I knew ultimately that Isaiah would have to wean himself from the breathing assistance and would have to have a good heart rate without the steady medication and sedatives, so I wanted to see Isaiah try and honestly felt that lowering doses and ventilator pressures would help.

The nurses and doctors, however, would disagree. Sometimes I wondered if it was because they didn't want to hear the buzzers, or if they really cared. I was conflicted because I knew they cared, but I guess I just wanted them to push Isaiah a little more. I tried to stay in the NICU for hours at a time monitoring his progress so the nurses wouldn't increase the ventilator pressure or the sedatives, but I knew I had to let go physically and let God spiritually do His own work.

Trusting God seemed one of the hardest things to do, but I knew I had to. For the sake of Isaiah, Jelan, my career and the rest of my life, I was about to make a choice that could affect my family's future forever.

~~~~~~~~~~~~~~~~~~~~**5**~~~~~~~~~~~~~~~~~~~

THE DECISION

"All this also comes from the Lord Almighty, wonderful in counsel and magnificent in wisdom."

Isaiah 28:29

I GLANCED INTO Isaiah's eyes as he stared through the large plastic incubator at his momma. It had been about a month, and his sweet, soft skin was brightening as his energy appeared at its best. He was still breathing with a ventilator and still needed quite a few sedatives and blood transfusions, but Mommy's baby was growing!

My daily routine for 28 days had been to wake up at the house, say a prayer, grab a snack and head three blocks to my baby's assigned spot in the NICU. Isaiah and I would read books, and depending on the nurse and the risk of infection, I could hold him and hum sweet songs. I loved watching that kid watch me, and I believe he grew fonder of the ear phones that played the classical music that scientists have predicted for years would make children smarter. I still think Isaiah enjoyed the upbeat gospel tunes a little more than he did the classical, though, because it appeared the beeping sound that alerted his low heart rates or fast-paced breathing were more quiet when the music played. The hospital in which we were based was within a large medical university, so a music therapy student tapped on quickly to Isaiah's love for her singing and guitar skills. Their bond went so well that they considered using Isaiah in a study to detect which type sounds were most beneficial for a premature child.

The Experiments

The decision to allow Isaiah a slot in the wide pool of scientific experiments at the hospital became easier as I learned to accept the fact my child was not a study rat but maybe a breakthrough in the medical realm of cures for other premature babies. Everything from my child's urine to his blood and even his X-rays and glucose levels were tested regularly and documented in students' journals. In addition to these studies, my laid-back spirit also resulted in Isaiah becoming the spectacle of the visiting middle school and high school students who came to the NICU to write their own reports. Many of them could hardly believe such a tiny body held a living soul.

I learned later that I was also able to decide which nurses would oversee my child. Of course, I picked a short, loving nurse name Amanda who had just married but had loved on little NICU babies for years. I also selected a couple others: Tamara, who was pregnant but drew me because of her matter-of-fact points of view, and Nancy, a red-headed woman who had also had a premature child some years ago. But these type choices, from the music and the nurses, were miniscule compared to the one I was about to make – whether or not to return to work after my six weeks of maternal leave and few days of vacation.

Thinking Things Through

I had sought every possible avenue with the corporation that managed our company's leave to stay longer. However, without medical documentation that I suffered some psychological or physical disability that prevented me from working, I would have to return to the office in just a few days or risk losing my position and my job altogether.

Other mothers and fathers at the house had been tasked with the same decisions. Some quit and left their jobs and all other stability they knew for the sake of their children. Some faked they were losing their minds (so they say they faked) and were given extra days off. Others recognized what little stability they had as necessary for their child, so they found ways to get back and forth from wherever they lived as often as possible to be with their little one. There was no public transportation from my town to the hospital Isaiah was in but I had recently gotten a new vehicle, so had we a need to travel back and forth, then we could.

As far as the psychological option, I called my gynecologist's office and expressed my misery. One of the nurses recommended I go to a local emergency room, but that the medical personnel would likely keep me there for 10 days for a psychological evaluation. That turned into a non-option because I was trying to gain more days with my child, not less for being cooped up in a hospital room. So my soul remained torn as the decision involved more than just me. It included the rest of my family, and especially Jelan.

I masked my frustration to friends and co-workers in e-mails like this one, which was around a week before my scheduled return:

May 18, 2009
Subject: Isaiah a Month Old!

Hey folks! Mr. Isaiah pulled in strong this month, weighing 2 pounds and 2 ounces today :). He is eating like a horse and keeps his eyes open for longer periods of time.
It appears everything he is going through is typical of a premature child, and there is nothing that should spark a major concern. The brain bleed is not getting any worse, thank God, and we are still trusting it will be totally resolved by the time he is ready to come home. Doctors say his release date will depend on him, though we are trusting he will be home by August, when he was due. There is no weight requirement for him to come home, but he needs to be able to breathe well, continue to eat well and have stable organs (and be big enough for my sitter not to be scared to break him :).
Mommy is good, too. I'm continuing to trust God and trying to stay focused. The medical folks are suggesting (not yet mandating) I rest a few more weeks beyond the usual 6-week leave and return mid to late June, but I miss you folks so much.

I may be one of few who runs to work to keep me sane instead of running away from it.
Thanks for continuing to keep us in your prayers.
Much love

I figured that somehow God would see fit to grant me more time to stay with my child. I didn't know what to do anymore, and the decision was one friends and families refused to offer an official suggestion for.

Luckily, I walked into the NICU that day and found my child off the ventilator and on a new continuous positive airway pressure (CPAP) machine that doctors were testing in hopes of weaning him and other infants off of the ventilator. The CPAP machine worked like the ventilator in some ways but allowed him to do more work with his own breathing, versus forcing the breathing through his lungs. Isaiah didn't do so well, though, so they put him right back on that lung-blowing machine. His toes were completely blackened, but a plastic surgeon believed the cells weren't totally dead and could possibly return to normal. I looked over the full length of Isaiah's body and thought of healing scriptures from the book of Isaiah in the Bible.

Isaiah's Point of View

There was a nurse there who allowed me to hold Isaiah's hand. I told my baby I wouldn't burden him with my problems because I knew he was going through a lot, but I wanted to know how he felt if Momma would have to leave. Those who have never been in my situation might have called this verbal transaction with a minimally responsive child senile. For me, it was therapy. It seemed as if Isaiah was saying through the fewer beeps from the ventilator that he would be alright, but that he wanted me there. As I held my baby's hand I remembered the first day doctors said we wouldn't end up where we were. They thought he wouldn't make it, but he had lived at least a full month. Then he was breathing on his own, although they came back and said that he couldn't. A test from his lung secretions had shown that he suffered from bacteria known as ureaplasma. The bacterium was not potentially fatal, but it did seal a fate of future respiratory problems for some of the babies.

But there were the other breakthroughs, like when he stopped needing the blood transfusions. And there was the first time I got to hold him, or listen to his heartbeat. There were the times I laughed with the respiratory therapist about what sports he would play, or the moments I would have to call the doctor to ask some one-on-one questions. It was the breakthrough moments when I first held his little hand, or the time he moved his miniature toes. So many memories had developed beside his bedside. The thought he wouldn't fully recover within the few days in which I would have to leave the big city was almost too much to handle.

I felt absolutely miserable that day. I had held a plush turtle that I won at a support group close to my bosom so it would carry my scent, and I laid it beside him. I told him Mommy still had a few days to think, but that I would spend fewer hours with him over the next week and leave "Mr. Speedy" there in absence just in case I decided to go back home. If he did well with Mr. Speedy, then maybe he would be okay if Momma went home to make a living. If he didn't, my weird logic told me I would have to give up my job and move up to the city where Isaiah was to be near. Jelan would have to stay with family while he edged toward his first year of school, and I would have to rush Isaiah to health.

Even the Smallest Miracle Counts

Isaiah did no better or worse with Mr. Speedy there over the first couple days of the week, but I walked into a surprise a couple days before I had to make the decision on whether to leave. He was off of the ventilator and back onto a CPAP machine, which meant he was breathing better and not suffering as much damage to his lung tissue. Then, another breakthrough came. A hospital that was only about an hour and a half away from my home that didn't accept highly sick babies could actually accept Isaiah once he started breathing better. So if I decided to go to work, I could still drive the distance to see Isaiah every day versus rare and far between in the hospital he was in at the time. Some nurses urged me to take the move for Isaiah into consideration, while other nurses believed it was in my baby's best interest to have his mom there.

Isaiah was two pounds and five ounces, which was a full pound more than when he was born. He liked to move his head and his feet. He had no heart problems and the brain bleed was continuing to dissolve.

Prayer unearthed that for me, stability was much more functional if I returned to work, visited Isaiah on the weekends until the transport to the other hospital, and stayed near my then 4-year-old Jelan. So, the decision was finally made.

I kissed my finger and placed it on Isaiah's hand. I braced myself and gathered all the numbers I needed to call every few hours to check on my child. Then, with tears in my eyes and a voice strained with pain, I told Isaiah goodbye at his fifth week of life and made my way back to my home.

~~~~~~~~~~~~~~~~~~~~**6**~~~~~~~~~~~~~~~~~~

CLOSER HOME

"Lord, you establish peace for us; all that we have accomplished you have done for us."

<div align="right">

Isaiah 26:12

</div>

I FAITHFULLY VISITED Isaiah every weekend after I had left the hospital and was proud to report more stories of progress each time. I had followed pounds and ounces to the tee while I was at the hospital, only to notice that he seemed to grow even more while I was gone. He certainly ate more, and at around two months of age, we started experimenting with a bottle. My little guy did very well, though he tired sometimes and would have to be fed by a tube again (it was some time that I would squeeze the milk out on the towel so he would not be responsible for as much. It seemed he was overfed, anyway). Still, he kept his eyes open more and was weaned from CPAP to an incubator that had an "oxygen environment." This allowed a nurse to monitor how much oxygen Isaiah was getting but it didn't require him to wear any sort of breathing apparatus. He had gotten thick enough to wear clothes, too, so I was able to bring him some warm blankets and sweet little outfits from home.

The greatest news I had received in a while came while I was on a week-long business trip in California. Isaiah was doing so well that he was finally able to move closer to my family, which meant that for the one weekend I was about to miss from the weeklong trip, someone would be able to drive the hour distance to see my son. Many from the family would get to see Isaiah for the first time since he was born! I tried to get a flight out earlier than initial plans but couldn't. It was okay though. I would see my baby soon in an area I knew better than the gargantuan facility in which he had lived since birth.

I would soon realize that the care from such a large hospital was second to none, however, as I watched my child take a couple steps back because of lesser equipment at the new hospital and fewer nurses who knew him personally. The new hospital did not have Oxygen environments so Isaiah would have to go back to a nasal cannula that helped him breathe. He went back to full tube feedings because he didn't want to eat. He awoke less often. Perhaps the worst of it all for me, though, was the inability to call over the phone to check on my child while I was in California because one of the nurses had forgotten to give me some secret code. The nurse refused to tell me whether the child was dead or alive. I went through a mental imbalance as all I could do was focus on the three-and-a-half-hour flight back to my child.

When I got there I didn't want to see him with the grief I had in my heart until I talked to someone in charge. The person didn't really seem to understand my concern and gave some explanation on how the hospital was looking out for my child. I wanted to make a written report, but I didn't have the nurse's full name who would not tell me about my child. I inquired about transferring my child back to the other hospital but knew that insurance likely wouldn't buy my reasons why. So, I calmed myself down, washed my hands and found a hospital gown in order to see my symbol of light in his new surroundings.

A New Place to Stay

He was beautiful. As my grandmother said, Isaiah had "filled in" and was no longer skin and bones. His plush cheeks were the rosy way I imagined a newborn child's cheeks I had seen in the pictures, and his black hair was curling. He had on a little white t-shirt and a diaper for children from zero to five pounds. In the back of my mind, I could picture an angel a little bigger than him watching my little boy sleep. The image reminded me that whether I was nearby or far away, Isaiah was trying his hardest to get better so that he could come home. And God was watching over him as he did it.

With him only an hour way, I was able to review his progress in person at least twice a week instead of just once, and I didn't have to pay for a room to stay as often as I had in the other city because we were so much closer. I was given a code to call and to come in and see Isaiah whenever I wanted, and sometimes I would sleep in the NICU waiting room just to wake up to his beautiful face.

I don't know how time flew so fast, but it seemed like hours instead of months that had passed between when I had first left Isaiah in June until August, when my four-year-old was preparing for school. This reminded me more than any other time that my decision to return was the best choice for my family, because both my sons were able to have their mother in some capacity. Jelan had trouble adjusting in school at first. I didn't know if it was because he didn't get as much attention from Mommy as he had expected or if he was just not ready for the change, but I tried my best to make the relationship between the two brothers as smooth as possible. My plans were somewhat complicated when swine flu, a deadly and feverish virus, broke out throughout the country and the hospital prevented children Jelan's age and younger from visiting. It became yet another task to explain to him that he couldn't see his brother until the little one came home, but we were able to make it through.

Another Ride

I borrowed some more of Jelan's books and continued to read and play Isaiah music. He continued to strengthen and started back opening his eyes. I could hold him more and tell him how much his family loved him, and I was able to read the Book of Isaiah for longer periods of time because it seemed like he was actually listening. He started drinking almost all the milk placed in the bottle, though he still needed to strengthen his jaws so he could suck for longer periods of time. Things went very, very well for a couple more weeks.

And then Isaiah just stopped breathing.

The nurse called me while I was on my way to another reporting assignment to let me know that doctors pulled out every breathing trick they could to bring my baby back to life. While Isaiah finally came back, we started back at Zero as far as needing a ventilator to breathe. His heart rate was dropping more often. Tubes were inserted for antibiotics and the blood transfusions became a possibility again. He couldn't wear clothes for a few days and they stopped feeding him altogether. I began to thank God that Isaiah was closer to home because I don't know that I could have driven as fast as I did the distance to the other hospital without wrecking. Yet, that day was the first time I prayed that God take my baby away so he wouldn't suffer anymore, especially if that were to be the ultimate plan. I was trying to accept things as they were, and in the meantime lost most all the hope I had maintained throughout the last couple months.

I began to come to conclusions of him parting life or not being able to live the normal life we had hoped for. If Isaiah wasn't going to be able to see after suffering retinopathy of prematurity, which was a disconnection of the blood vessels behind his eyes, then I hoped he could at least hear. If his toes were to fall off, then at least he would still have his arms. If he couldn't breathe alone, at least he could eat. I knew the thoughts reflected almost as little faith as I had the day my water broke, but I was weakening and was trying to find the strength not to give in completely.

Apparently, no one told Isaiah that Mommy was trying to give in. Doctors determined that he might have had a seizure that caused him to stop breathing, so they placed him on some medicine and watched to see if he would bounce back. He trudged along, and eventually started back breathing – almost on his own! He gained weight back and was soon able to start eating from a bottle again. He was back on the clock of the hospital that required all its babies to go at least a week without any heart rate drops or breathing difficulties before coming home. My God, how grateful I was to see his recovery closer to home as nurses asked me to leave and "refresh" my spirit. Isaiah could tell when I was stressed, they said, and the last thing he needed was for the main support system he knew to become overwhelmed.

I apologized to my baby for underestimating his ability and took the short trip home, praying all the while that my baby would soon call "home" the same place that I did. I was trying to mentally get closer to my spiritual home, too.

~~~~~~~~~~~~~~~~~~~~~**7**~~~~~~~~~~~~~~~~~

A CALMER STORM

*"...for in perfect faithfulness you have done marvelous things, things
planned long ago. ...Surely this is our God; we trusted in him, and he
saved us. This is the Lord, we trusted in him; let us rejoice and be glad in
his salvation ...Trust in the Lord forever, for the Lord, the Lord, is the
Rock eternal."*

Isaiah 25:1, 9, 26:4

AFTER TWENTY-THREE weeks and one day I got yet another
call. This time, evidence of months of prayer finally surfaced.
Nurses from the hospital were wondering what day of the week I
could come and spend the night at the hospital so that doctors
could monitor my care for my son. I knew from experience with
Jelan that this meant Isaiah was coming home!

I booked the very next day to attend Cardiopulmonary
Resuscitation, or common CPR courses, as well as other parenting
classes so the hospital could release my baby to me.

Doctors were still a little concerned that Isaiah was not
eating as much as he should have. We contemplated the possibility
of a G-Tube inserted through his stomach so he could process his
food, but the surgery would have to be done at Isaiah's previous
hospital. I declined because I believed that once Isaiah was home –
our home – then he would do better. My hypothesis would prove
correct. I stayed the necessary one night to prove I could care for

my own child, and the next morning, my baby was in a car seat and headed to our house!

There was no need for any oxygen but I was given plenty of handout information on what to do in case he stopped breathing. The little brown car seat we purchased matched his brown and cream outfit, and the tiger on his shirt was certainly exemplary of the fight he had to endure. He was around eight pounds when he finally took what we hoped would be his last trip from a hospital.

While Isaiah didn't have to come home on any oxygen, he still was a heavy breather because of all the scarred lung tissue he had. He had to take breathing treatments, and he slept somewhat lightly. We had a home in the country so he was able to get some of the best air because of all of the surrounding trees, and although I was skeptical of germs, he was able to have many, many more visitors than were at the hospitals with him.

I still played his music, as we weren't completely out of the woods. Isaiah would face the likelihood of some defects like cerebral palsy and an attention deficit disorder, and would likely be behind schedule in most everything from crawling to eating solid food. It was the possibility that his eyes would weaken because of the ROP, but doctors had said it was just shy of a miracle that he could see at all. He tested positive for a genetic deficiency that would make him allergic to certain foods, and he was to follow up every few months at the hospital four hours away for doctors to detect any learning disabilities. He had bronchopulmonary dysplasia, which doctors predicted would cause rapid breathing and other lung difficulties for some time. The blackened tips of his toes had fallen off, so some of the toes were shorter than the others on one foot. It was likely he would continue having seizures.

Regardless, as I looked at Isaiah on our own couch versus a hospital's, he looked back, and it was almost as if he had smiled. His curly hair was covered with a hat in the fall, and his little feet had on socks for the first time. He was able to see his brother after more than a month of isolation and soon, he was able to sleep in his own bed.

Of course, I still hadn't learned with his birth what it was like to hold a healthy newborn baby. The records were proof he had suffered a long while. The medications were real, and it was highly probable that there would be even more storms ahead.

But for the time being, the storm had calmed, and my son could break from his battle in his own home, in his own mother's arms. The scripture I had held so tightly to – Isaiah 53:5 – had come to fruition. God was a healer, and the proof was in Isaiah's first chapter of life.

CONCLUSION

"Surely he took up our infirmities and carried our sorrows, yet we considered him stricken by God, smitten by him, and afflicted. But he was pierced for our transgressions, he was crushed for our iniquities; the punishment that brought us peace was upon him, and by his wounds we are healed."

Isaiah 53:4-5

AS PAINFUL AS some sections were in this book, I have an overall peace and settling joy for the opportunity to share my baby's life with the world. Isaiah is truly a remarkable child, and because of his willingness and strength at times I felt that mine was sucked away, he survived as one of few 23 weekers doctors said could live. I truly believe miracles played a part, because the worst of what doctors expected seemed to lose against Isaiah in the months after he came home.

Isaiah had three stays in local hospitals for pneumonia in his first year because his lungs had not fully developed. It was often he had to return to oxygen, and he was diagnosed with mild cerebral palsy. However, the seizures subsided and doctors noted no dysfunctions in his brain. Isaiah was slow to speak and to move, but at around 15 months, he had started scooting and was proficient in the words "DaDa" and "Hi." He got his first haircut at age one. He loves to wrap his mouth around one's lips in a slobbery kiss, and with a combination of speech, occupational and physical therapy through an early intervention program, he is catching up well with everything else.

While Isaiah has been diagnosed with cerebral palsy, the only visible sign is that he wears braces to keep his balance. Thankfully, he is expected to come out of those in a few months from this book being published.

I truly appreciate your interest in Isaiah's life and your support of research into prematurity altogether. I pray that God grant your family peace if you are going through a similar trial, and that he grant you sincere thankfulness if you've not experienced our saga but have wonderful and healthy children. Please don't hesitate to recommend Isaiah's Chapter to others who may be experiencing or already have endured the roller coaster of a NICU.

PHOTOGRAPHS

Isaiah was born at 23 weeks, one day gestation in Birmingham, Alabama. He was one pound, five ounces. In this photograph (lower right), he is approximately one month old. Nurses allowed me to hold him for a few minutes at a time so he could feel my heartbeat. He still needed a ventilator and a feeding tube.

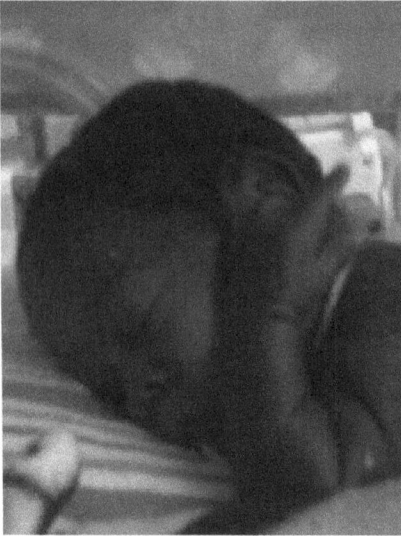

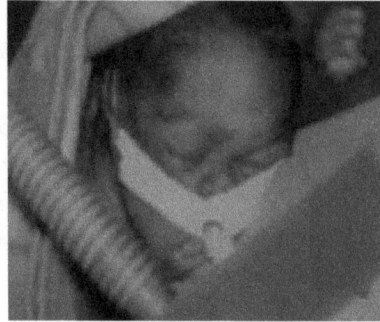

Below, Isaiah is about two months and still in need of the ventilator. Monitors are placed on his back and a small blood pressure cup on his tiny arm.

Above, Isaiah takes a break from most of his cords and the equipment in preparation for a bath. The nurses were great with allowing a few photos in between his transitions.

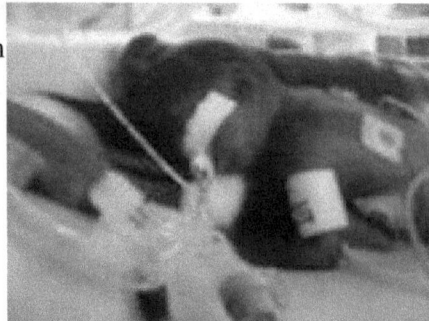

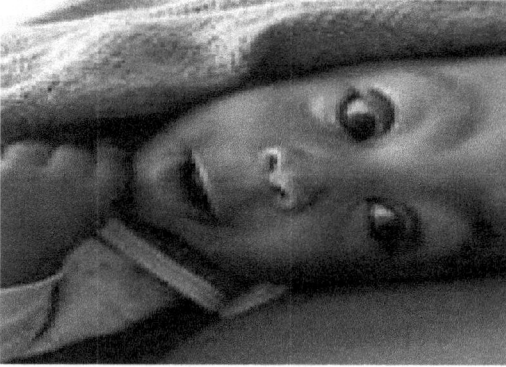

Words can't express the joy we finally experienced when Isaiah came home about five months after he was born. He's since been a happy, bubbly and outgoing child who is far from "normal," but more amazing than any child I could have prayed for. I pray one day he will share his own stories of courage and strength.

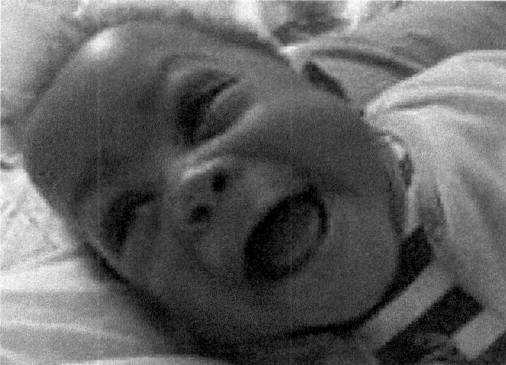

RECOMMENDED PRAYER

Dear Lord,

I know this is a trying time that you have seen before.
I know that my sweet baby is not first to take this climb.
And God, I can't explain how we have ended on this road,
but our prayer is you keep us and don't let us fall behind.

I know this little baby is an angel sent from Heaven.
I'm sure you see his pain and that he's fighting for His
life.
So Lord, I pray you carry him as he goes on this journey.
Please grant him peace and give us hope and stay here
as our guide.

And Lord, while I'm away from here and he just keeps on
growing,
I know that you will make a way and keep him safe from
harm.
I pray your love shines through the hands of all who
touch his body
until the day you bless me, Lord, to hold him in my arms.

Amen

RECOMMENDED RESOURCES

Below is a partial list of online resources for families who
have premature children, or people who are interested in learning
more about prematurity:

Kids Health: www.kidshealth.org

The March of Dimes: www.modimes.org

*U.S. National Library of Medicine on premature babies:
www.nlm.nih.gov/medlineplus/prematurebabies.html*

Parents of Premature Babies, Inc.: www.preemie-L.org

Premature Baby Premature Child: www.prematurity.org

Parents Helping Parents: www.php.com

Ebony Horton

ABOUT THE AUTHOR

Ebony Horton is an esteemed journalist, commentator and mentor with extensive experience in the southeastern region of the country. She has worked for *New York Times'* regional papers and has had published work appear on *USA Today*'s website. Ebony has edited books that are published in Christian and secular markets as well as served as an expert reviewer of short stories, essays and poems. She has an undergraduate degree in English and Master's Degree in Publishing. Her memberships and activities include community service at-large with Delta Sigma Theta Sorority, Inc., community sports and writing organizations, and her church, Northview Christian Church in Dothan, Alabama.

Books available at Amazon.com. For more ordering information or speaking engagements, contact Ebony Horton at ehortonedits@gmail.com.

www.ingramcontent.com/pod-product-compliance
Lightning Source LLC
Chambersburg PA
CBHW071439040426
42445CB00012BA/1398